An A-Z guide to getting older

A survival handbook

Eleanor Watkins

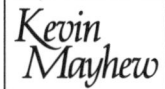

First published in 2002 by
KEVIN MAYHEW LTD
Buxhall, Stowmarket, Suffolk IP14 3BW
Email info@kevinmayhewltd.com

© 2002 Eleanor Watkins

The right of Eleanor Watkins to be identified as the author of this work has been asserted by her in accordance with the Copyright, Designs and Patents Act 1988.

All rights reserved.
No part of this publication may be reproduced, stored in a retrieval system, or transmitted, in any form or by any means, electronic, mechanical, photocopying, recording, or otherwise, without the prior written permission of the publisher.

9 8 7 6 5 4 3 2 1 0

ISBN 1 84003 890 X
Catalogue No. 1500496

Cover illustrations by Simon Smith
Cover design by Angela Selfe
Edited by Elisabeth Bates
Typeset by Louise Selfe
Printed in Great Britain

Ageing – a poem

When your hairline's receding,
   eyesight growing dim,
you need glasses for reading,
you're no longer slim;
when a brisk uphill walk
leaves you puffing and blowing,
and your joints tend to creak
as you're coming and going;
when your doctor and lawyer,
your dentist and vet
and the new sales assistant
who's rather a pet,
your boss and work colleagues,
your clergyman too,
well – everyone really
is younger than you;
when memory fails you,
your knees let you down,
high blood pressure ails you,
your brow shows a frown,
when your chinline is sagging,
your toes tend to gout,
your footsteps are lagging
where once you strode out;
when no one has kissed you
for days and for weeks,
when you suffer from wind
and embarrassing leaks,
when you have to watch diet
and take medication
and twelve kinds of tablet
on every vacation –
then, though it may cause you
to weep on my shoulder,
I have to inform you
that you're getting older!

A

Adjustment

Different types of people may face the onset of Senior Citizenship in different ways. You may be the kind who carries on just as before, with your work, your family commitments, your interests – hardly noticing that another big 0 has passed preceded by a higher digit. You may go into denial, with a colour-rinse, a trendy wardrobe and evasive tactics when your D.O.B. is called for. Or you may greet this part of your life with an ominous feeling of fear and dread.

However you approach it, some adjustment will be needed. You, or your husband, may be nearing retirement, or have reached it already. Your children will probably have left. Your energy may be a little less boundless and your metabolism slower. Your memory may play tricks on you.

Take heart. The golden years can be rich and fulfilling. Ways around problems can be found and age does have its consolations (more of that later). Best of all, God stays the same, and with each year that passes you are that much closer to that place with him where time is no more; there'll be no sadness or grief or parting, and you'll have seen the last of sagging jawlines, arthritic joints, thinning hair, and other woes of ageing you thought would never happen to you but did.

Adult children

Being parents is quite a different ball game when our children have passed the teen years, the student era, the moving out or starting a career or getting married stage and are adult people in their own right.

We may feel faintly astonished to find that we have raised these mature, decision-taking, responsibility-shouldering people who were once so dependent on us. It can be a poignant moment the first time we realise they're actually taking care of us rather than vice versa.

The relationship with our adult children will depend very much on the way we related to them in their growing-up years. Hopefully, our grown-up children will be among our closest friends. They'll need other friends, though, and so will we, so we must be careful not to monopolise their time and attention. And it's wise not to be too forthcoming with advice − unless, of course, it's asked for.

Advice

It can be tempting to carry on dishing out advice to your children in the way you've always done. Probably they resisted your advice in their growing years, though they may have relied upon it and taken it on board far more than you realised. As they got older they may have asked your opinions on things, and even acted upon your advice. It's rather a shock when you realise that your children are the experts now, and are advising you on where you should live or spend holidays, when you should retire, what kind of car to buy and products to use, etc. etc. (It's all for your own good, of course!)

This turning of the tables can provoke mixed reactions. It's rather touching that they care, but many of us feel we're not quite ready to give up all independence and freedom of choice just yet. However, most of us oldies are wily enough to be able to carry on doing what we want without upsetting our children too much, while letting them think we're following their advice. One of the nice things about being older is that younger people (not just our children) do seem to think that with our grey hairs comes extra wisdom, meriting a flattering measure of deference and respect. (And, hopefully, we have enough maturity not to let it go to our heads!)

Anniversaries

See also
Birthdays

There'll be more and more as the years pass. All the birthdays, wedding anniversaries, Mother's and Father's days, Christmases, Easter Days, and family high days and holidays – will be multiplied when your children furnish you with their spouses, in-laws, and, of course, your grandchildren. You will also probably have gathered many friends over the years.

I learned two things about remembering anniversaries from my mother-in-law, who is in her late 80s, has numerous friends all over the world, plus six children with spouses – eighteen grandchildren including spouses, and two great-grandchildren with three more expected soon.

1. Keep a calendar on the kitchen wall with names and dates.
2. Go in for bulk-buying of greetings cards.

B

Bed

See also
**Comfort,
King-size bed,
Nights, Sleep**

Bed can be an increasingly inviting place to be when you begin to feel the weight of advancing years. Not only is it a place to sleep (hopefully), it also is that comforting cosy haven where you read, write, watch TV, talk on the phone, have breakfast, or just enjoy a cuddle. There's something very appealing about climbing into your warm, comfortable, private sanctuary at the end of the day. Travel may be great fun, even when you're older, but there's nothing quite like getting home to your own bed.

Bereavement

See also,
**Death, Loss,
Regrets**

Bereavements will happen oftener as we get older. Most of us who still have parents living will have to face their loss sooner or later. The same with uncles and aunts. We will probably begin to value more those who are left as their numbers decrease. If we want to pick brains, gain insights into family traits and history, put right differences or make amends, better do it now while there's still time.

We may also notice that a disconcerting number of our own friends and contemporaries are leaving this life. It's a shock to realise that some of them are no age at all – in fact, they're our age!

It's hard to know sometimes how to deal with bereavement in others. We're often afraid

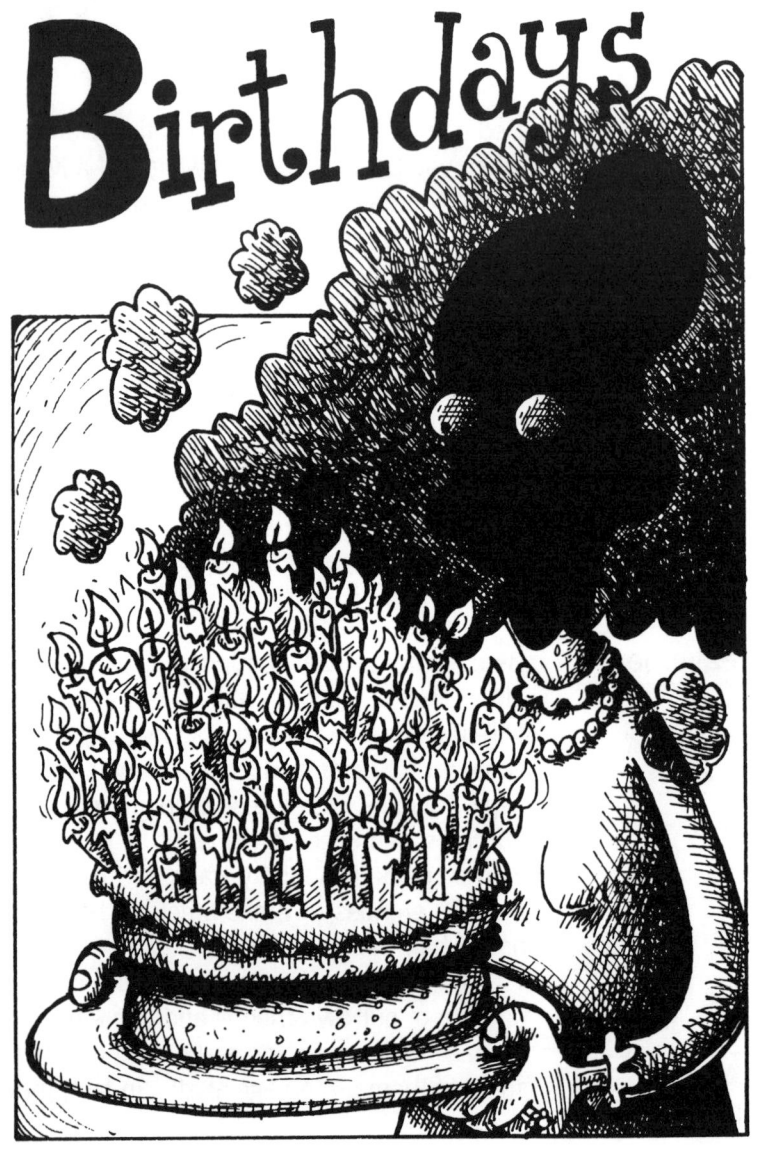

of saying the wrong things. Better, though, to take that chance (there's really no right thing to say) than say nothing at all. A word or two to show we care, reaching out with a hug or touch of the hand, may seem a small thing but mean a lot. As people progress through the various stages of bereavement, they often need to talk over the details of their loss and about their loved one, perhaps repeating the same things over and over. A listening ear and time to listen can help.

Bible Study

See also
Promises of God, Scriptures

One of the nicer things about being older is that we're likely to have more time for regular periods of Bible reading and study. There's also the advantage of being a little wiser and able to understand and appreciate scriptural truths and precepts, because we've tried and tested them in our own life and experience. There's great comfort in *knowing* (not just hoping) that God's word is absolutely to be trusted.

However old and wise we may be, we still need our regular daily intake of scriptural nourishment. And however long we've lived, there are still new and wonderful truths to be discovered as we study the Bible.

Birthdays

See also
Anniversaries, Time

Remember how we looked forward to our birthdays when we were children, and how long it seemed until the next one came round? We enjoyed our birthdays then, had great parties and boasted about the latest age we'd attained. Later, there were some significant birthdays, but in between we weren't really that keen on celebrating another year gone by. Until we reach senior citizenship. Then, suddenly, it becomes possible again to boast about our age (especially if people pretend they don't believe it!), celebrate with a lavish party and generally have fun. And they tend to come round much quicker than before, too!

Books

If, like me, you love books, you have a priceless treasure no one can take away from you. You may no longer be able to run a marathon, jog a couple of miles or even sprint for a bus, but you can enjoy reading as long as your mind holds out (and it'll hold out a lot longer if you exercise it with reading!). You may need stronger reading glasses, large-print books if your eyesight becomes very poor, but all these helps are there for the asking.

C

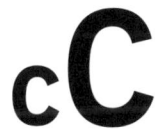

Changes

Changes come as we age, like it or not (and most of us don't).

Physically, our bodies slow down, wear down and sometimes let us down. Mentally it's the same story. But there's part of us that can't be changed by physical ageing, and only improves as time goes by. Our spirits are in God's hands, and will go on for eternity. God has guaranteed to change us into the kind of people he intended us to be, and he will work on us throughout our lifetimes to bring about that change. And one day, we will discard our worn out bodies and be clothed with glorious new ones that will last for ever (2 Corinthians 3:18).

Changing roles

See **Adult children, Relinquishment, Retirement**

Children

See also
**Adult children,
Family,
Grandchildren**

As we grow older and the rigours of our own child-rearing years slip into the background, many of us find a new appreciation for the company of children. Somehow, children become more precious, we recognise their individuality and potential, and also understand how quickly the years of childhood pass. When we're younger, and busy, there's often no time to sit and talk to a child and listen to their views of the world. We're often too involved with other things to take time out to look at things with a child – uncurling leaf-buds, baby animals, snowflakes and changing cloud patterns. I well remember taking a winter walk with my first grandchild, when she turned to me and said, 'Doesn't this mud feel lovely and squidgy under our boots!' It did!

One of the consolations of teetering on the brink of second childhood is that it's much easier to make friends with people who are still in their first.

Church

Church congregations are mainly made up of old ladies, or that's what popular opinion often tries to make us believe. Sometimes true, maybe, though not in the churches I go to. All the same, older ladies do form a significant part of a church family, and very valuable they are too. Who else could be relied upon to boil kettles, prepare teas, arrange flowers, organise events, mend furnishings, type up minutes, prepare copy for newsletters, open up premises, wash up, clear up, and do a million other essential things? Let's not forget, also, the input of wise counsel, listening ears, shared experience, encouragement and nurture that people of mature years can offer the younger ones in their church family. And let's all remember to show proper appreciation of our older members.

Clubs

In most areas there are lots of clubs catering for older people. Joining a club is an excellent way of meeting new friends, getting involved in the community and maybe learning new skills. It's also a good opportunity for sharing your faith with those who maybe wouldn't be comfortable in a church. You don't have to be ancient and decrepit to be part of a club for older people. I know a sprightly 71-year-old who looks about 50, cycles thirty miles without turning a hair, and gallivants about the country at the wheel of a mini-bus full of older people all having a jolly good time.

Comforts

See also
Bed, King-size bed, Routine

We like our comforts as we get older, and why not? We need warmth for our creaking joints, ease for aching limbs, peace and quiet for our frazzled nerves, a predictable routine for our slowing metabolism. We can do without those nasty shocks, unpredictable changes and stressful traumas that disturb our comfort. None of us like to be forcefully ejected from our nice cosy homes and predictable routines.

It doesn't hurt to be gently nudged out of our comfort zones every so often though. Like taking up new hobbies. A new sport, even. Going to new places. Or a mission or outreach project. Some retired friends of mine recently found themselves on a short mission trip to the mountains of Nepal, set off with grave misgivings and their own mountain of medication – and loved every minute. And they appreciated their home comforts even more when they got back to them.

Computers

See also
E-mail, Technology

Computers may seem to be a mysterious closed book to many older people, but it doesn't have to be that way. You may not be the Internet whizz-kid that your primary-age grandchild seems to be, but you too can learn. There are many excellent computer courses on offer at schools, libraries and colleges, available to all and beginning with the very basics. Being computer-literate can open up amazing new opportunities and widen horizons in this technological era, whatever your age. It's simpler than it seems!

Confidence

Our confidence does tend to dwindle as the years increase, not helped by dimmer eyesight, duller hearing, memories that play tricks or joints that seize up. The younger people are now the ones in the swim of things, and often we feel relegated to the sidelines of life. Remember, though, that our confidence is in God. He is the one who upholds and strengthens and enables us, who plans each day of our lives for us, and will be with us as we come to the end of our life here and step over into the next one.

Consolations

There are so many consolations and pleasures in later life that I've listed each under its own separate heading. Some older people lead such fulfilling and interesting lives that their only problem seems to be finding enough time to fit everything in.

See: Clubs, Computers, Exercise, Experience, Family, Food, Fun, Future, Grandchildren, Heaven, Holidays, Just the two of us again, Laughter, Memories, Old friends, Pensions, Promises of God, Retirement, Self-knowledge, Understanding, Wisdom.

Control

See also
**Dependency,
Independence,
Relinquishment**

There is a relinquishment of control that comes with the ageing process. Mercifully, it usually doesn't happen all at once. But sooner or later, former things, or at least some of them, come to an end or diminish, from holding down a responsible job or raising a family or both, through to eventually perhaps having to be cared for by others.

Giving up control of our lives doesn't come easy. Yet, for the Christian it's one more step in the yielding of ourselves into the loving hands of God. Ultimately, our Father God is in control of our whole lifespan, and we can rest secure in that knowledge.

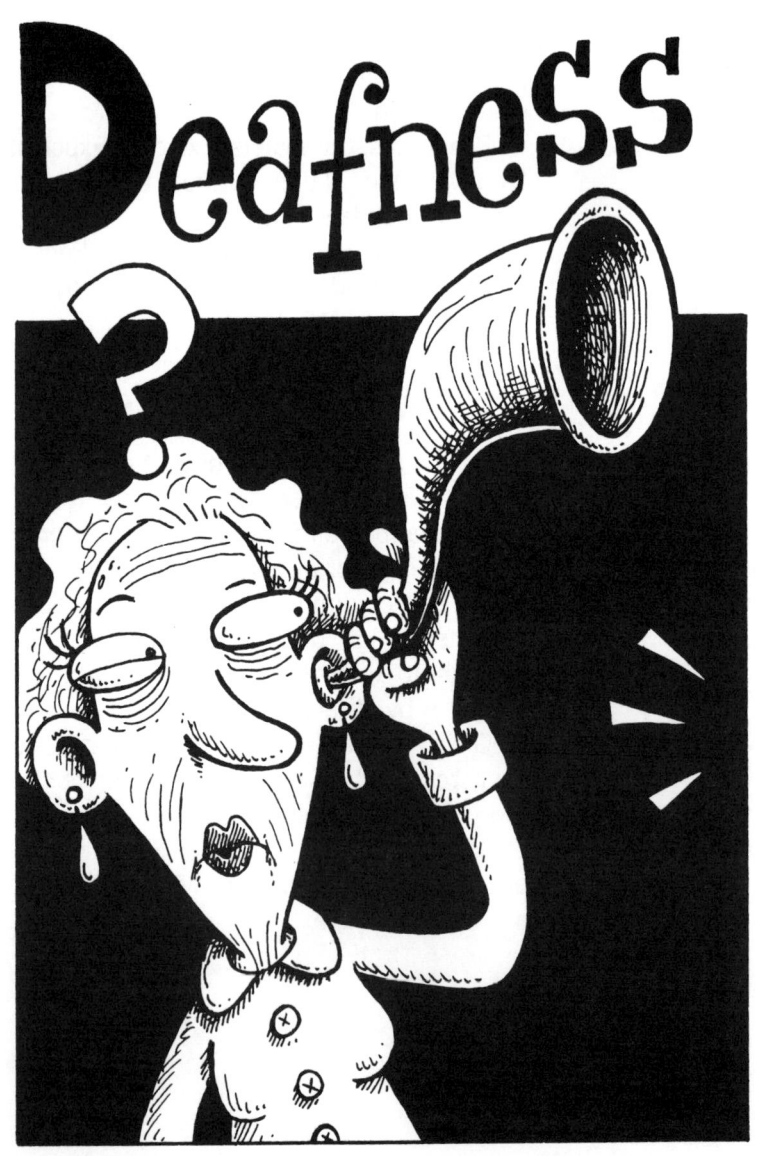

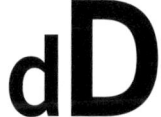

Deafness

Most people get a bit hard of hearing as they get older. It can be quite tempting, when this stage is reached, to be conveniently deaf when you don't want to hear. The downside to this is that others might call your bluff, and you may hear a few things about yourself that you'd rather not.

Seriously, if your hearing is causing problems, see your doctor. Modern hearing aids are small and discreet, and usually very efficient.

Death

See also
Bereavement, Loss

Death (whether your own or that of someone close to you) is something most of us would rather not dwell upon. When we're younger we tend to feel it will never happen to us, but there's no avoiding it really. Thankfully, none of us knows exactly when we will die. That's in God's hands and we can safely leave it to him. It's the great unknown, and the God who sees us safely through the changing experiences of life will surely see us through this one – which, after all, is not an ending but a beginning of a glorious new future with him that will never come to an end.

Dentures

There are advantages to wearing dentures.

1. You don't get toothache.
2. You can always get a new set when these wear out.
3. Children are impressed by your ability to wiggle them about and take them out.

There can be problems with dentures. A friend of mine was in hospital and on the first morning a trainee nurse collected the dentures of the elderly patients for cleaning. The problem was she put them all into the same bowl . . .

Dependency

See also
**Independence,
Relinquishment**

We don't like to be dependent on others, do we? Most of us will struggle to do things for ourselves as long as we possibly can. It's not the end of the world to be helped by others though. Most people in the caring professions are just that – caring, and they're well trained in what they do. I know people who have wonderful friendships with their carers, and carers who are blessed and encouraged by the faith and the personalities of the people they care for.

Depression

A state of mild chronic depression is more common among people of middle-age and beyond than they might like to admit. Let's face it, if we listed depressing things that happen there'd be a long list.

True clinical depression – the sort that means you can't carry on the normal activities of life – needs medical treatment and shouldn't be accepted as hopeless. There are all kinds of treatments and therapies that should sort out even severe depression.

For that mild, debilitating sense of apathy, boredom, ennui, discouragement and general lowness of spirits, you may need to take a firm line with yourself. However you feel, whatever you do, don't just vegetate in front of the TV set. Decide you're going to change. Find a new interest or hobby, get out and about, maybe take a trip or a holiday. Learn something new – whether it's computer technology or line dancing or whatever. Reach out to others with a letter or visit or phone call. Ask someone to pray with you – or better still, join a prayer group. Take long walks in the countryside. Get a pet. The possibilities are endless. Above all, don't consign yourself to the scrap heap because that is definitely not where you belong.

Doctors

As we age, we will get to know our doctor better – mainly because we'll spend more time in his or her consulting room. It's important to have a good relationship with our doctor; to be able to speak freely and trust we'll be understood. Anyone of any age is at liberty to change their doctor if they're not happy with the one they've got. It's not being disloyal. Or if they'd rather see another of the practice doctors – for instance, one of the other sex – then that's their right and privilege too.

Driving

It's one of those inevitable facts of life that as we age, not only do the policemen get younger, but so do practically all the other drivers and road-users. They also seem to get much faster and more unpredictable; there are more of them and they are definitely more lacking in patience when we dither at road junctions, peer shortsightedly at road signs, cause a 2-mile tailback as we cruise comfortably at 40mph, or absentmindedly indicate left when we intended to turn right.

eE

E-mail

See also
**Computers,
Technology**

If you have access to a computer, e-mail is an excellent way of keeping in touch. E-mailing is fun! Letters take time to arrive and chatty phone calls can be expensive. But with e-mail (especially if you take advantage of the free-time offers) you can have instant, bang-up-to-date contact with friends and family anywhere in the world. Especially good for communicating with distant grandchildren – they'll be computer literate from early on and will be impressed that you made the effort to learn too!

Empty nest

See also
**Just the two of us
again**

An empty nest seems like a strangely barren, lonely, echoing place when the last child finally leaves, with his or her accompanying belongings, clutter, mess, noise and friends.

But you'll adjust very soon, and in no time you'll appreciate the blissful quiet, the freedom, space, neatness and privacy. You'll find, though, that the children will descend on you for visits or to stay, and will inevitably bring with them friends, fiancés, spouses, children and pets . . .

It's good to see them and even better when they leave and you get back your lovely tranquillity, privacy and peace.

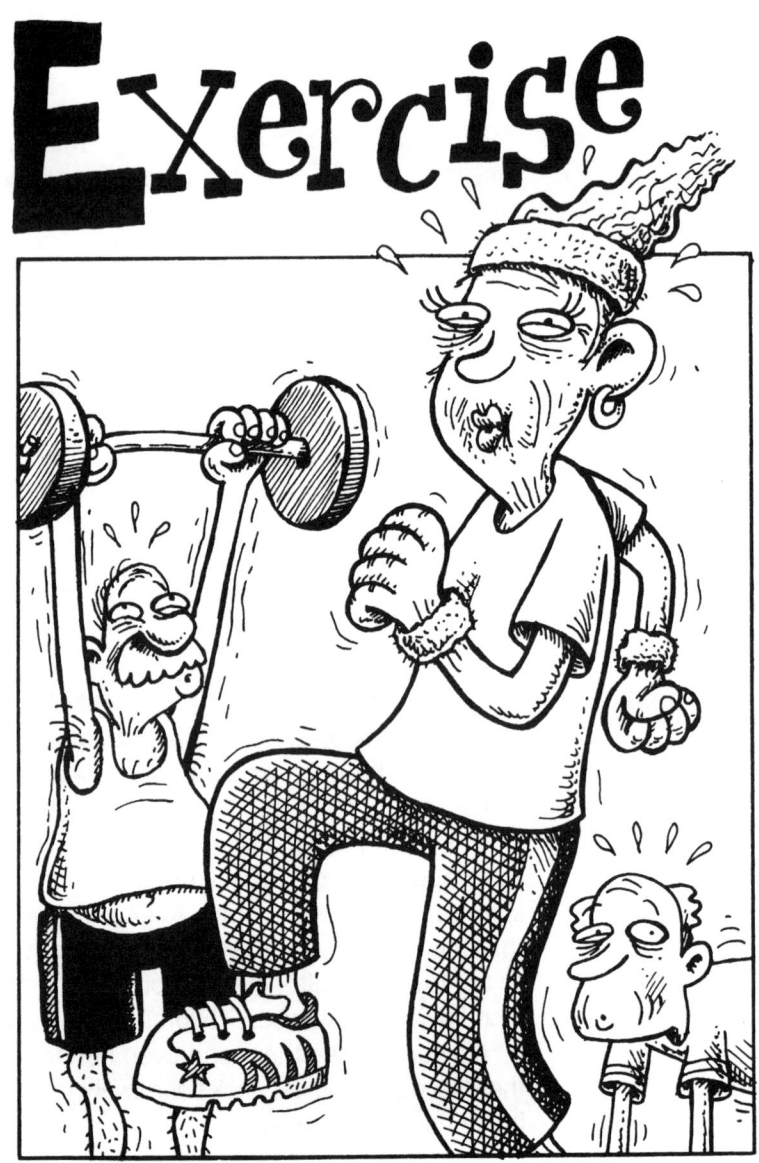

Energy

Your energy levels will drop as your body ages, your metabolism changes and everything slows down. This may be frustrating if the rest of you is still raring to go!

Getting enough rest is important, as is a good balanced diet and plenty of exercise. A doctor friend of mine swears by taking a little nap after lunch every day – just 10 or 15 minutes, but it's enough to get batteries recharged for the rest of the day.

Exercise

Exercise is a must if you are not to seize up, stiffen up, fatten up and eventually give up. Ideally, exercise should be a habit that starts in youth and carries on through middle-age and beyond, maybe adapting as the years roll by. Even the most dedicated couch-potato can benefit from beginning to exercise, though a doctor should be consulted about the way to tackle it if you're planning to start something new. It doesn't have to be drastically energetic or something to endure. Swimming, cycling and dancing are all excellent ways of burning up calories and loosening up joints, and walking is maybe the best exercise of all and available to almost everyone.

Experience

'Putting it down to experience' is a wise maxim and one that works if we are willing to learn from our experiences, and go on learning. We'll never attain perfect wisdom in this life, but we can be teachable and humble even in later years. We may be able to share some of what we learn with younger people, though there are many things they can only learn through their own experience. As we get older, it does appear that even the seeming disasters of life are often turned round to bring a greater good, for ourselves and for others. Most of all, over the years we learn that though all else may fail, God is faithful (1 Corinthians 10:13).

Eyesight

See also
Glasses

Eye checks are important – vision changes as we age. Reading glasses that were right last year may need to be changed for stronger ones now. After around 40, most people grow long-sighted, but this may change again later on. Your optician can also detect at an early stage the onset of conditions like cataracts or glaucoma, and prescribe the appropriate treatment.

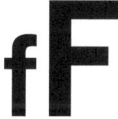

Family

See also
**Adult children,
Grandchildren**

Families are funny things, and in some ways get a little trickier as time goes by. For example, more family members will be gathered along the way as children, and nieces and nephews, acquire partners and in-laws, who all meet and interact from time to time.

It's hard enough, with our memories not what they were, to remember who's related to whom, or whose aunt or uncle this may be, or who has recently lost a loved one – even putting a name to a face is sometimes hard.

It's lovely, though, when we meet someone new – a nephew's girlfriend, etc. – and find we really click with them.

Fashion

To those who have understood and appreciated the freedom it brings, growing older can be a truly liberating experience. No longer do we need to slavishly keep up with the latest trends or fashions. We have probably learned to know ourselves very well, have the maturity to know what suits us and what we're comfortable with, and the courage to stick to our guns.

Food

Whatever you eat, after middle age, it tends to settle around the waistline and hips. This is unwelcome but true.

Food becomes more of an issue when you're older. I remember the days of feeding a growing family, when you bought in bulk, planned out meals well in advance, cooked and served up whatever you decided was wholesome, nourishing and filling, at the double.

Suddenly, you're shopping and cooking for two again and the whole thing can become much more of a big deal. It can take ages, wandering round the supermarket, to decide whether you fancy a bit of fish or a chicken breast for dinner tomorrow. Or which brand of marmalade is most tasty. Or which cereal is less likely to cause indigestion, or whether that label of coffee will keep you awake all night...

Eating out is hazardous because you never know what stuff they're putting in the sauce. Eating out in the evening means you'll be up half the night. Eating at your children's means you have to pretend you like those herbs and garlic they use to flavour everything. Eating out at picnics and barbecues is risky because of the insects that might get in the food. Eating at home is the safest option – if you can just decide whether you fancy a nice chop or a bit of gammon.

Forgiveness

See also
Regrets

Getting older can often bring a more reflective frame of mind, which can include looking back and taking stock of the years that have passed. Often old hurts and grievances will surface, maybe things that we thought had ceased to trouble us. It's good to take a little time to face things as honestly as we can, maybe with a trusted Christian friend or prayer partner, to make sure there is no buried resentment or bitterness that has not been dealt with. Unforgiveness tends to bring with it a host of other ills that prevent our enjoyment of life. We can't always forgive in our own strength, but if we face things as honestly as we can and ask for God's help, he will enable us to forgive, and to know the freedom that forgiveness brings.

Fun

You don't stop having fun the minute the first grey hair appears or you get your first pension book. In fact, maybe now's the time to bring a little more relaxation into your life, especially if you've reached retirement. Make a positive plan to include 'fun' in your calendar – whether it's something as exciting as planning an overseas trip, or something as ordinary as eating out or exploring your own neighbourhood.

Future

There is always a future to look forward to, no matter what our age, status or situation. Whatever has happened to us during our lives, however sick and frail our bodies, each day brings new possibilities and God will keep us securely in his care. Beyond that, we can look forward to a glorious eternity, with wonderful new bodies and a loving Father who himself will wipe away all tears and fill us with his perfect joy (Revelation 21:4).

Glasses

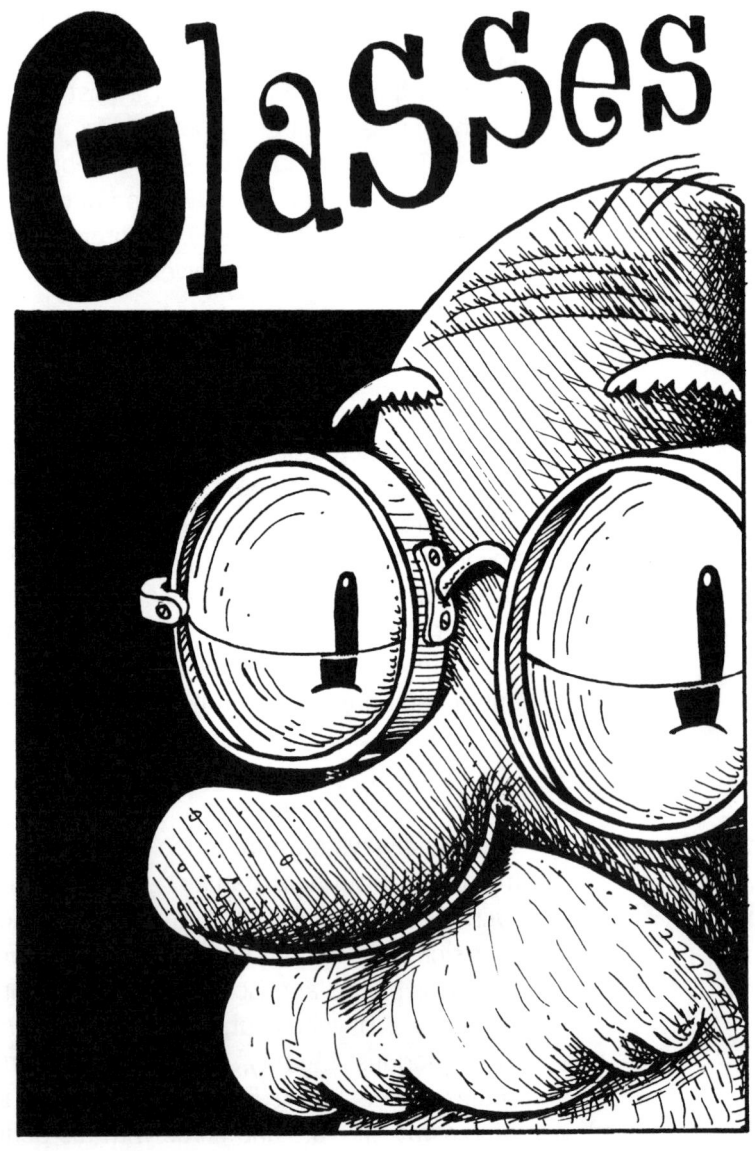

gG

Generation gap

In some ways, we oldies will differ from the younger generation, in others we are remarkably similar. After all, we've experienced most of what our descendents are going through, and a bit more. Times are different, true, but human nature remains much the same. Most younger people are prepared to listen to what we have to say, especially if we resist the temptation to bang on too much about what things were like in 'our day'.

Glasses

See also
Eyesight

Reading glasses are a necessity for most people after about the early or mid-40s, when the eyes change and become long-sighted. You realise the situation when you have to hold your book further away to get the focus right.

The need for glasses heralds a whole new way of life. A great deal of time and effort will be spent putting them on and taking them off, cleaning and polishing them, remembering to take them with you and, especially, looking for them when you can't remember where you put them down (a pity that failing sight and loss of memory happen at about the same time).

Just the same, glasses are a wonderful invention and enable us to keep on doing the things we want to do, so we can thank God for them.

God

Most of us who are Christians will sometimes wonder just exactly what he's like, this God we belong to and whom we seek to love and serve. The first disciples asked the very same things: 'Who is God?' 'What is he like?'

The reply that Jesus gave was simple and to the point. He simply stated that anyone who had seen him (Jesus) had also seen God the Father.

We can do no better than read the Gospel accounts of the life of Jesus to learn about the character and nature of our God.

Grandchildren

I think I would put grandchildren right at the top of a list of consolations of later life. Until you have them, you may be slightly mystified or bored (or a little envious) of hearing of the delights of grandparent status from others. When you get your first grandchild, you'll understand exactly what they're on about.

Having grandchildren is like having children all over again, but better. This time you get to enjoy the fun and games, the high days and holidays, the silly jokes, the spoiling and the outings and the dressing up – and when it's time for the dull stuff like nappy changing, clearing up, enforcing rules and routines and being responsible – voila, the parents take over!

With grandchildren, you relive that keen delight in seeing the world and everything in it for the first time. You have the joy of knowing that you are a unique and special person to your small grandson or granddaughter. You can even boast about your grandchildren and get away with it!

There's another side, though. You'll soon learn that if your grandchild is ill, or hurt, or distressed, you'll suffer every bit as much as you did with your own children. But hopefully you'll have the advantage of perspective to help you and enable you to help the parents and the rest of the family.

Gravity (law of)

All of us on this earth are subject to the law of gravity. I remember being taught in school science that, apart from this law, we'd float to the ceiling, or take off like a released gas-filled balloon.

As we get older, the law of gravity kicks in with new meaning. Gradually, our bodies (or relevant bits of them) begin to drop, sag, droop, fall out and generally head downward.

Take heart. We're daily getting nearer the time when gravity will cease to trouble us, our bodies will change and we'll rise to meet our Lord in the air (1 Thessalonians 4:16-17).

Greying

The particular time our hair turns grey seems to be something of a lottery – some people begin to grey in their 20s or 30s, some hardly change hair colour at all. A friend of mine died in her 70s with never a grey thread in her beautiful dark hair. Most fall somewhere in between.

Heredity probably plays a significant part, and there's really no pill or potion available to stop it happening.

We can cover up the grey hairs if we wish, of course – it's entirely our own choice. If you feel better with a colour rinse, then rinse away, or if you choose to, stay grey. Take comfort from the dignity and respect that the Scriptures afford those who have achieved the dignity of grey hair (1 Timothy 5:1).

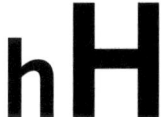

Health

See also
Deafness, Doctors, Eyesight

Health checks are very important when we are growing older, no matter how fit we feel or how well we have looked after ourselves. As we age, our bodies slow down and work less efficiently. We can prolong our fitness and activity by paying attention to such aspects as diet and weight, exercise and sleep and proper checks. We must take notice when our bodies tell us that something may be wrong, or simply that we cannot expect to perform as we did twenty or thirty years ago. We don't want to turn into chronic hypochondriacs, but we mustn't neglect ourselves either. Our bodies are still the temples of the Holy Spirit, and as such must be respected and cared for. Don't be tempted to skip medical, dental, ophthalmic, chiropody or any other service available. You're fully entitled, as a Senior Citizen, to free health care.

Hearing

See **Deafness**

Heaven

Revelation 21
That's where we're heading, and what a glorious future awaits us! Gone will be our ageing bodies, our aches and pains, our strivings, frustrations and limitations, our heartaches, disappointments, and all the other negative things that

frustrate and spoil our time here on earth. There we will meet again those we loved who have gone before. There we will no longer 'see darkly' but understand at last the wonderful mysteries of God and eternity.

We are not given much advance information of what Heaven will be like – maybe our limited human minds could not take in the wonders awaiting us.

But we know that we will see our Lord Jesus face to face, that we will be with him for ever, and even that he himself will wipe the last of the human tears away from our eyes (Revelation 21:4).

Holidays

The time when our children have left home and are on their own can be wonderfully liberating for parents taking their holidays. Suddenly there's no need to consider what the younger ones will want to do or where they will want to go. Now you can please yourselves again, book a cosy small cottage or apartment instead of a family one, afford a flight or a cruise that you couldn't with kids in tow, or even go cycling or back-packing if you want to and are fit enough. (Kids do these things too but wouldn't dream of doing them with parents.) Don't feel guilty about the freedom and space you now have – you deserve it. Accept those long-standing invitations to visit friends abroad, seize any opportunities that come your way – and enjoy them!

Holy Spirit

John 14:16-17

The Holy Spirit comes into our lives to befriend, empower, help, comfort, guide and instruct us, and the aim of all this is to conform us to the likeness of Jesus. This work is not done in an instant, but will go on until the end of our lives. So we will go on growing and changing, however old we are. We will change, but the Holy Spirit will not.

The Holy Spirit is the spirit of Jesus, who will indwell and fill a person who has received Christ. With his help, we can do the work that God has prepared for us, whatever our age. God has promised that he will pour out his spirit on everyone who will receive him, young and old alike (Joel 2:28-29).

Home

We all find ourselves with more time at home as we get older, especially when we or our spouses, or both, reach retirement. Some of us may move house around then, maybe opting for something smaller or easier to maintain, or nearer to amenities or family members. Some adult children may be over-zealous in wanting to have us where they can 'keep an eye on us' – very nice, and lovely that they care, but don't feel pressured into making a move until you are ready.

Now can be an enjoyable time in home-making, with both sharing things like redesigning, decorating and gardening.

AN A-Z GUIDE TO GETTING OLDER

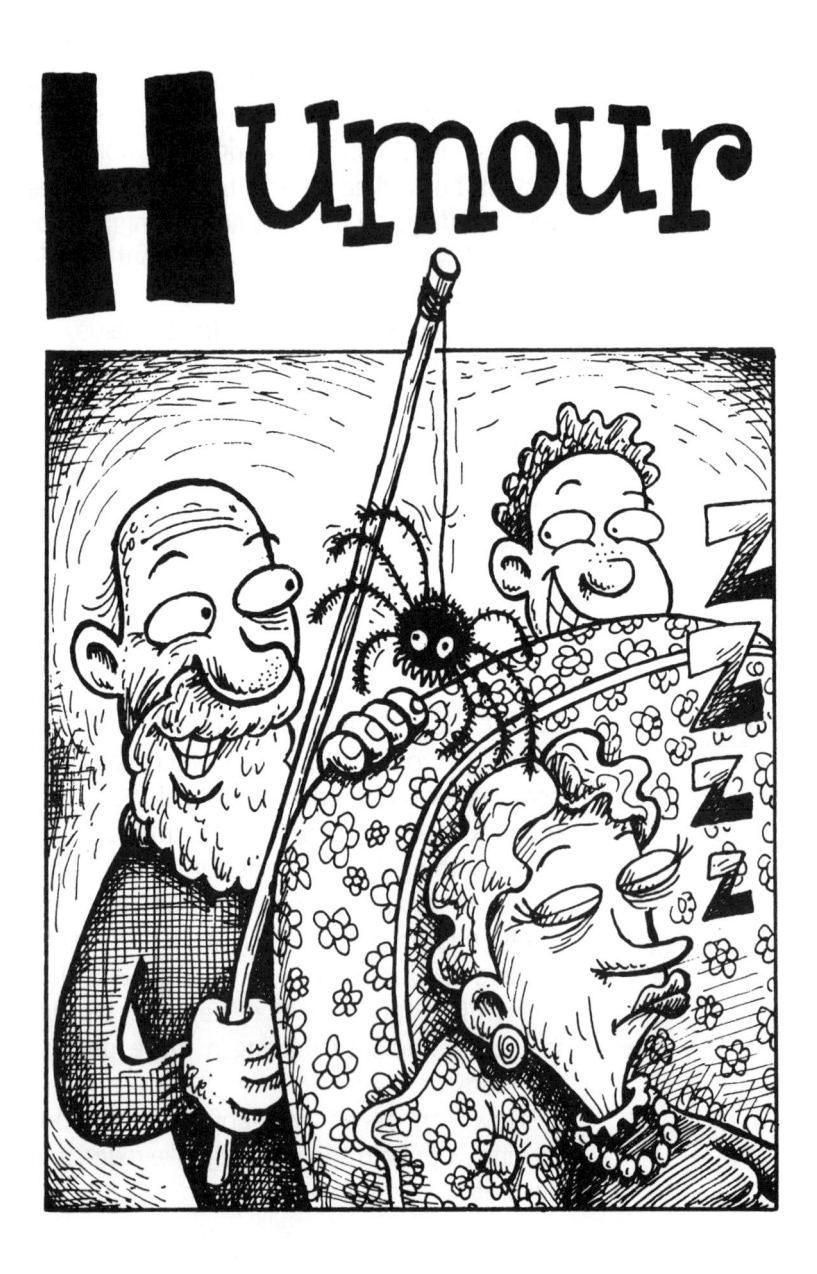

Humour

Hospitality

Hospitality is something that almost everyone can practise, and it's something that God approves of (Romans 12:13).

Older people maybe have a greater opportunity to use the ministry of hospitality, when work and family no longer claim so much attention. It doesn't have to be elaborate. God can bless the simplest action (Matthew 10:42).

And your house doesn't have to be like something out of *Ideal Home*! A cup of tea, a meal, a bed for the night or few days – all these can be immeasurable blessings if they're offered with a warm welcome, listening ear and attitude of love. God can use our homes in wonderful ways, whatever our circumstances, whatever our age.

Humour
See also **Laughter**

If you're blessed with a good sense of humour it will stand you in good stead as you get older. Humour can take the sting out of situations that could lower the spirits and get you down. A sense of the ridiculous will tide you over many an embarrassing scenario.

We don't all have the same sense of humour, but all can help to lighten life, unless we're having a laugh at the expense of others. That's just negative and cruel. But if we have the ability to laugh at ourselves we have a great advantage, and one that can be shared.

A humourless elderly person is off-putting, but people naturally gravitate to one who laughs and looks on the bright side.

Illness

See **Doctors, Health**

Independence

See *also*
Dependency, In-laws, Limitations, Relinquishment

The giving up of even a degree of our independence comes hard to us all, and most of us will struggle to retain our independent status as long as we possibly can. This is fine when we're fit and healthy, especially if we're half of a couple. For people growing older on their own, it's wise to have a means of alerting a friend or neighbour if something is wrong; for instance, if a fall or accident happens and it's impossible to reach the phone. An agreement with a neighbour to call, or keep a lookout for telltale signs like milk bottles not taken in or curtains left drawn may be reassuring. Alarms to be worn round the neck are useful, but many people don't like wearing them or forget to put them on. Someone local popping in for a quick visit on a daily basis is maybe the best option for a frail person living alone. And it's a good idea to leave a spare key with someone trustworthy.

In-laws

With today's longer life expectancy, it's possible that some of us will have parents or in-laws still alive when we reach retirement age ourselves.

This can be increasingly difficult for those taking the role of carer, and not just in the sense that anything physical becomes harder, and that we risk injury to ourselves if we have to do heavy lifting or carrying. People in later old age often undergo changes in brain function, which may turn a formerly sweet-natured and reasonable person into a bad-tempered, fault-finding one. If this happens, try not to take it personally. Senility and dementia are real problems, and help should be sought before the carer feels overwhelmed themselves. However much we wish to fulfil our responsibilities, it's much harder for us to care for a parent or in-law in these circumstances than for a trained nurse or carer who is not emotionally involved. Much better to stay close, visit often and maintain a good relationship than struggle to do the impossible. Some families, of course, cope well and happily. But don't feel guilty if you can't.

Internet

See **Computers, E-mail**

jJ

Jesus

Our relationship with Jesus Christ is what matters more than anything else in our lives. Jesus is God's son who came to live a human life and then die a cruel death to take the punishment for our sins. To all who receive him he gives forgiveness and the right to be called sons of God, with a place awaiting them in Heaven after this life.

Nobody is too old to make their commitment to Jesus Christ, whatever kind of life they may have led, or whatever they may have believed previously. Jesus will lovingly receive each one who comes to him, making them into new creations, and will never leave them or forsake them (Romans 8:38-39).

Joints

As we age, our joints will stiffen, creak and generally protest when we use them. We'll probably notice it most when we get out of bed in the morning, or get up from a chair after sitting, after strenuous exercise or bending and stretching. Arthritis may or may not be present, but we should seek medical advice if we suspect it – for instance, if hips or knees become very painful. Whatever the cause, we need to keep as mobile as we can. Limbs and joints should be kept warm, and any strenuous exercise prepared for by doing gentle limbering up exercises beforehand.

Journalising

See also
Books, Writing

Journalising or keeping a diary of events is a habit best started long before old age sets in. It's a fascinating way of recording events, setting down our ideas and feelings as we grow and change, and charting the progress of our families and of the world around us. It's also an invaluable way of keeping track of just what happened and when – as we get older our memories do tend to play us tricks and can't always be relied upon.

Keeping a journal is a wonderful help towards maintaining mental activity, planning our futures, and disciplining ourselves to write something every day, or every few days. It will also provide a written record of family life that will be appreciated by children and grandchildren.

Joy

John 16:24

It may be hard sometimes to feel joyful, especially when circumstances seem against us or disaster hits. Let's remember, though, that joy is God's gift, one of the fruits of the Holy Spirit, and can stay with us whatever our age or problems. Human happiness is fleeting, it comes and goes, but the deep joy God gives will stay for ever (Psalm 16:11).

Just the two of us again

This can be a most rewarding time, with the kids grown and flown, and retirement here. Time to do now those things you've always hankered after (or some of them.) Many couples discover a new spontaneity in their relationship, or deep satisfaction in taking a once-in-a-lifetime trip, or some other project that could never be done when work and family had to be considered.

Even the simplest of things – like shopping and preparing a meal together, planning and planting a new flower bed or patio, taking day trips or caring for a pet can bring huge pleasure when there are just the two of you again.

kK

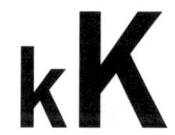

King-size bed

See also
Bed, Nights, Sleep

A new bed is a good investment as you begin to get older. For one thing, many couples may have slept on the same one for many years, and may not have noticed that the springs are wearing and the mattress sagging – not a good recipe for comfort when your joints and bones need proper support.

Now is a good time to consider a larger bed. One with two zip-linked mattresses is especially good: you can maintain your togetherness while not disturbing your partner if you toss and turn, or have to get up in the night, or rearrange your pillows, or decide you need a cup of tea – or any of the other things that tend to disturb our sleep when we're a little older.

King-size bed

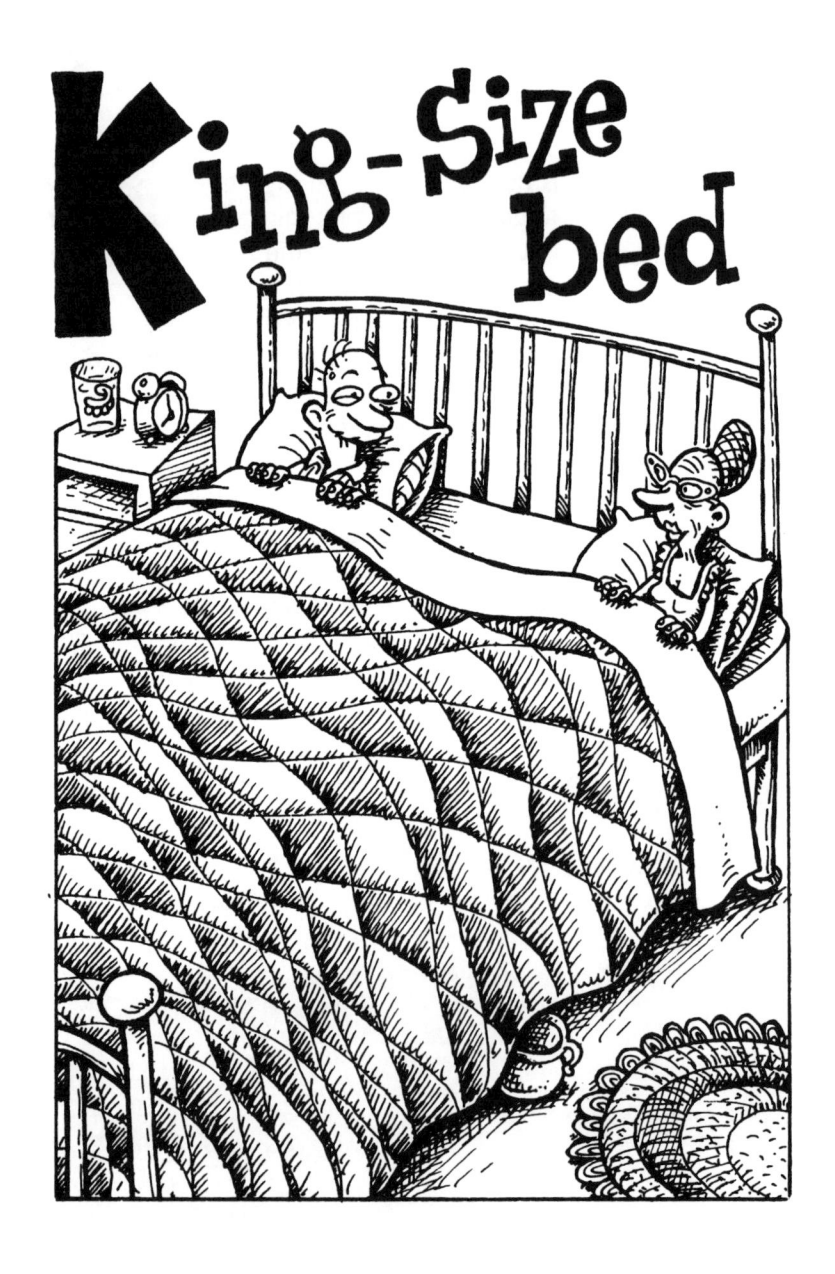

L

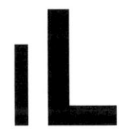

Laughter

See also **Humour**

Proverbs 17:22

A good laugh does us all the world of good – it's medically proven, as well as Scriptural. I work in a Christian centre where there's often a lot of laughter. The other week a whole tableful of older women were convulsed with laughter over some advice offered to one of them. Looking at them, I realised that four out of the five were widowed and that all had been suffering from varying degrees of depression and sadness. The following week they all said how much better they'd felt for that good laugh.

Our senses of humour may be different, but they're God given, and yet more evidence of his love and provision for us.

Limitations

See also
**Dependency,
Independence,
Loss,
Relinquishment,**

Limitations do happen as we age. The most obvious will be physical, a certain wear and tear on our joints and movable bits. That doesn't mean we should give up everything active – generally speaking, the longer we keep using our faculties the longer we'll keep them. But we'll need to use our common sense, too, and not put intolerable strain on anything to prove our point.

Our eyesight and/or hearing will probably need a little help. Mentally, there's no need to assume we'll deteriorate, as long as there's no underlying illness. Spiritually we won't age at all – that's one part of us that will keep on growing and expanding and developing as we stay in touch with God, to the end of this life and beyond.

Loneliness

Older people can be lonely, but then so can middle-aged and young ones. There's usually a certain emptiness when children leave home, and a much greater one when a spouse dies after a long marriage. A church fellowship and friends can do much to stand in the gap. But not all older people living alone are lonely – many appreciate the freedom and lead full and rewarding lives. Lone senior citizens are often a great source of strength, comfort and friendship to each other – meeting for coffee or lunch, sharing lifts, shopping, outings and activities. Many older people form the bedrock of voluntary staff in charity shops and find great companionship and satisfaction this way, as do the myriad of church workers and helpers who are older.

Loss

Losses of various kinds are part of the ageing experience. On a personal level, we'll lose varying amounts of hair, teeth, eyesight and hearing, bone density, agility, speed and brain cells! Many of these can be replaced with the help of medical science and technology, and most can be compensated for or dealt with in some way – even older human beings are quite resilient and adaptable.

There'll be other losses – of surviving parents, uncles and aunts, a spouse or partner, our jobs as we reach retirement, old friends as some of them die. Often we'll lose some of our income, maybe move house or district.

But there are gains too. With age comes experience, and experience properly used can bring a wisdom and serenity that is invaluable in helping those who are younger and less mature. We can gain enormously in our trust in God as we look back at his dealings with us throughout our lives.

mM

Making love

The intimate side of marriage can enter into one of its most rewarding stages as we grow older. Maybe we're slowing down a bit and don't feel like it as often as we used to. Maybe we have a few more aches and pains, stiffnesses and strains that make us a little less eager for the physical stuff. All this is OK and quite normal – as long as both partners feel the same and are happy with the status quo. If one is not happy with things as they are, some communication is needed. Don't be tempted to feel rejected and retreat into a silent huff, or, even worse, opt for separate bedrooms. Talk it through. And pray.

There are advantages to a later love life. There's more time to discuss how you're thinking and feeling. The need for contraception will be a thing of the past. If you're retired, you don't have to get up early. And you won't get kids bursting in at intimate moments, or teenagers phoning to be picked up at 2am.

Marriage

Because we have reached our Silver, Ruby, or even Golden wedding doesn't mean we can take our marriage for granted and not bother to work at it any more. A good, solid, loving lasting marriage relationship is one of God's most precious gifts and needs to be nurtured and appreciated, maybe even more as the kids leave and we find ourselves a couple again.

Some who have lost marriage partners may be contemplating taking the plunge into a second marriage, sometimes rather to their own surprise! A mature, second marriage can work very well and be one of the great delights and rewards of later life.

Medication

See also
Doctors, Health

Most of us will find ourselves in need of some kind of medication as we age. Some of us seem to need whole bags of things to keep us in good working order.

Some people find this a cause for anxiety and hold the rather puritan view that pills and potions are bad for us or habit forming. Let's thank God for his provision for us through medical science, follow the advice of the physicians (getting a second opinion if we feel we need to) and take whatever we need to restore our good health and well-being. It's all free after retirement age.

Mellowing

See also
Querulousness

We do change as we age, some of us mellowing while others grow grumpy and cantankerous. Having God at the centre of our lives will help us grow old gracefully more than anything, knowing that he will care for us at every age and stage of our growth.

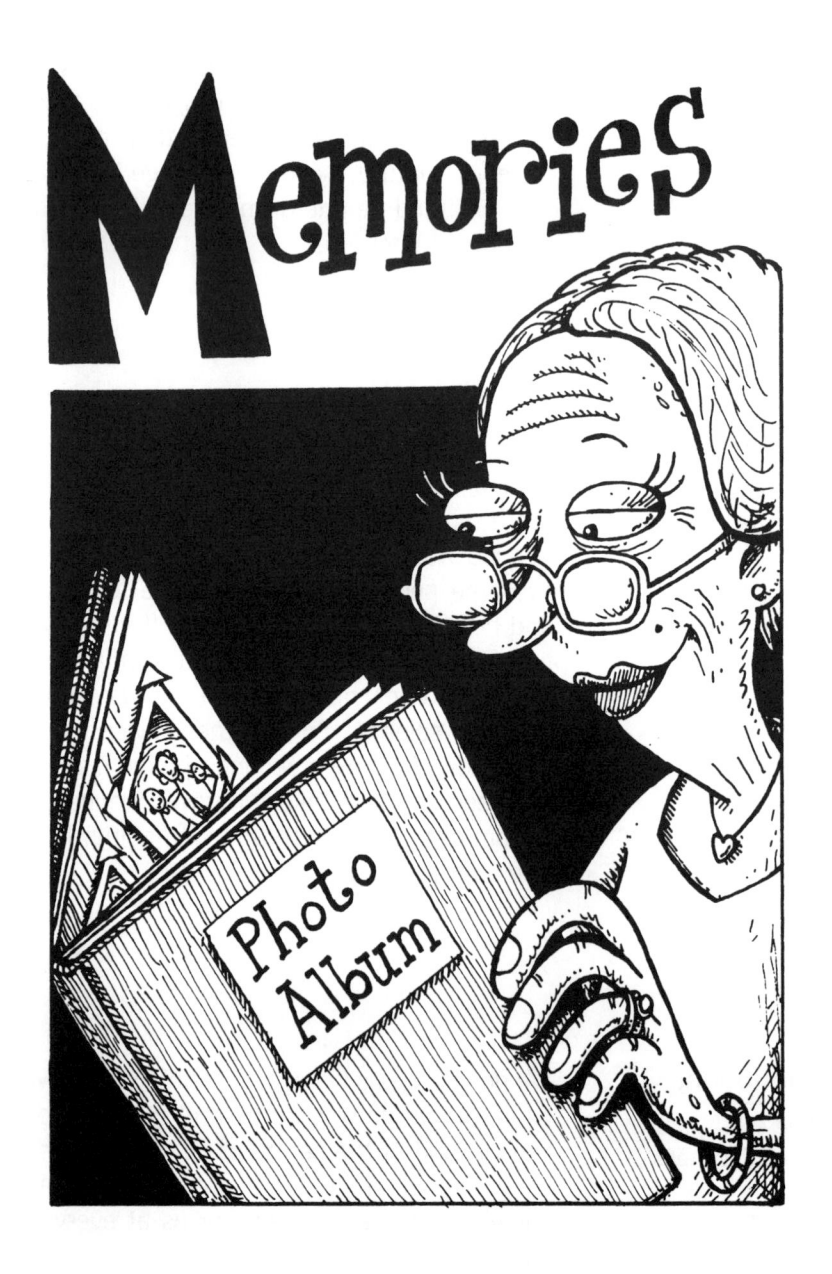

Memories

Memories

See also
Nostalgia

There'll be many precious memories to look back on as we enter our golden years. The events of past years do seem to take on a rosy glow as we recollect them, and it's great fun to gently reminisce with someone of the same vintage.

Quite often, our children and grandchildren are interested in hearing about 'the olden days' too – especially as time goes by and they realise that the older family members are an important link to the past.

Don't be tempted to live too much in the past, or over-romanticise the good old days. There were good and bad times then, as now.

Whatever our age, the present is to be savoured and enjoyed, and the future looked forward to.

Memory (loss of)

Why is it that we can remember exact conversations and sequences of events from thirty or forty years ago, while try as we might we can't recall what we had for dinner yesterday?

It's been rather depressingly explained that as our brain cells die off, layers of recent memory are removed, exposing the distant ones. None of this is cheering information.

Our brains are quite cunning, though, and can compensate for the memory loss by finding a roundabout route to what we're trying to recall. It takes a little more time, but gets there in the end.

Mirrors

After a certain age, mirrors are best dispensed with, or a least positioned in a dim corner or under a flattering soft light. That is the conclusion I came to recently when I was placed under a bright white light in front of a mirror at the hairdresser's. Prolonged peering into the mirror is definitely the prerogative of the young, fresh-faced and wrinkle-free.

Mobile phones

See also
Technology

We may not like the mobile phone, or the fact that every child, teenager, and far too many drivers seem to have one permanently clamped to their ear. They are expensive to use and there's a big question mark concerning health risks. We managed perfectly well without them in our day, didn't we?

However, if we can't beat them we may as well join them. A portable phone could be a real lifeline for an older person who needs to contact someone fast, whether at home or out and about.

Money

See also
Pensions, Wills

As Christians we may think it's all right to sail through life without a care, trusting God to provide for us in our old age. This may be a debatable point.

There will inevitably be a drop in income on retirement, whether or not we depend on a state pension. It's wise to discuss options and make some plans – not just about money, but about housing, possible moves, the eventuality of being left alone, illness, and so on.

It's not showing a lack of trust in God to do this. He expects us to make decisions for ourselves, with his guidance, as we did when we were younger, and this may include private pension or investment plans.

N

Negatives

There can be a tendency in older people to view life in a negative way. We all know those who seem unable to do anything but complain, relate their grievances, discuss their illnesses and look on the black side. (Negative thinking isn't confined to older people of course.)

As Christians, we need to remind ourselves of the long years when God has kept and blessed us, of his provision for us here and now, and of his promises for a future with him that will never end.

Nights

See also
Bed, King-size bed, Sleep

Nights ought to be peaceful in later life, with crying babies, sick children, straying teenagers and work worries well behind us.

Unfortunately, a new crop of sleep-defying trials seem to appear, from aches and pains, snoring and coughing and the need to spend a penny at intervals to the tossings and turnings of a spouse with the same problems. Just as well we don't need as much sleep as we did when we were younger.

Nostalgia

See also
Memories

Things were good in the old days, weren't they? The summers were sunnier, the winters snowier and the pace of life slower; people were nicer and children behaved better. And we managed without such things as microwaves, computers, digital cameras, videos or mobile phones.

Let's be balanced, though, and count the blessings we have today – health care, state benefits, social service support, counselling, better communications – to name but a few. We've probably seen more change in our lifetimes than in any comparable span of history. Let's be thankful for the past and enjoy the benefits of living today.

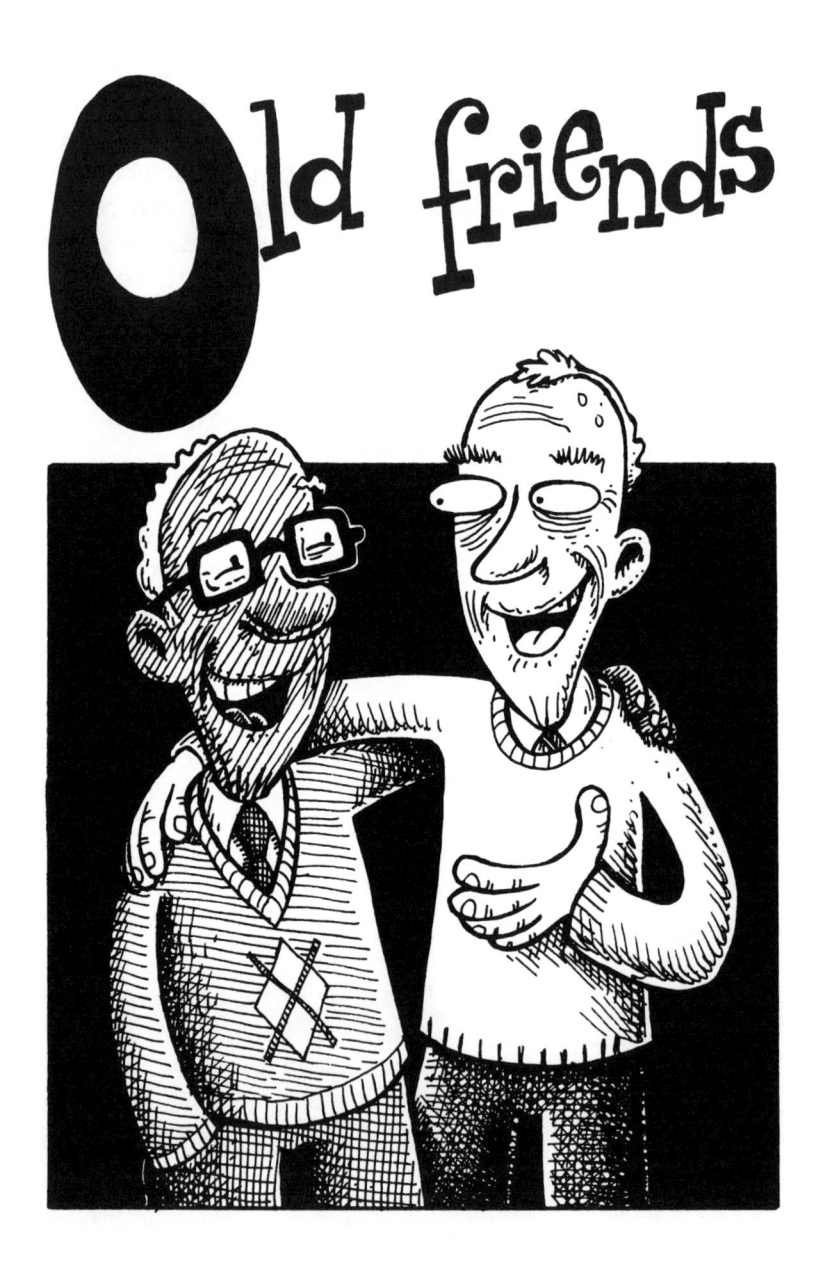

Old friends

O

Old age

The Bible has lots to say about old age. In both Old and New Testament times and culture, older people were cared for and respected (Leviticus 19:32; 1 Timothy 5:1).

Senior members of the family were honoured and valued for their wisdom and experience.

Things may be a little different in our day and age. Maybe we're tempted sometimes to question whether or not we have a place in today's society. Perhaps we need to remind ourselves that the most important part of us (our spirit), will never age, but will be renewed continually, as we stay close to our Father God (Isaiah 40:31).

Old friends

See also
Bereavement, Loss

Some of them go back a long way. A friend whom we've known from childhood or youth, through all the ups and downs of life, is a precious thing. Inevitably, sooner or later we'll experience the poignancy of parting with some of these as we all grow older. Let's value all our friends, old and new, enjoy them and let them know how much we appreciate them, while we're still on this earth together.

P

Patience

Patience does not automatically come with age. Some older people may have learned the lessons of waiting quietly and bearing with difficulties, but others certainly haven't. We all know Senior Citizens who are impatient, cranky and awkward.

Patience is one of the fruits of the Holy Spirit, and is cultivated by spending much time in God's presence, in reading his word and being in the company of his people.

Pensions

See also
Money, Wills

All of us in the UK, at 60 for a woman or 65 for a man, are entitled to receive the basic state pension with accompanying benefits (free medical prescriptions, travel and other concessions, winter heating allowance, etc.). There are additional benefits for those in special need.

It's sensible to think about supplementary provision for later life before we reach retirement age, whether or not we have additional pension schemes or income. Planning our finances is not showing a lack of faith, just practical common sense. Proper planning is also helpful to our children who may carry responsibility for our future.

Perseverance

See **Prevailing prayers**

Perspective

Our lives and times do take on a new perspective as we grow older, especially if God is at the centre of our lives. We may look back and wonder at the angst and heart-searching we went through over issues that now don't seem very important at all. We may marvel at the ways God has worked in our various situations, doing 'exceedingly abundantly more than we could ask or think'. We can be thankful for the hand of God upon our lives, and from this perspective we can take courage and trust him for the future.

Pets

Our pets are precious, especially if our families are a long way away or if we live alone. It's generally acknowledged that people with pets will be healthier and more stable and balanced, and even live longer. A cat is maybe the least trouble for someone less active, though dogs are excellent motivators for getting fresh air and exercise. Even a budgie or a goldfish will provide lots of beneficial interest and stimulus.

Plans

See also **Future**

Even though we're older and maybe retired, God still has plans for us. And they're good plans!

We may not be quite as much at the hub of things as we were (from the world's point of view) but God most definitely has plans for us for each day of our lives.

What security to know that our work, and the strength to do it, is all in the loving provision of our Heavenly Father.

Possessions

See also
Simplicity

Material posessions seem to lose their attraction, to some extent, as we grow older. Maybe we realise that we have a houseful of stuff we don't use or appreciate so much any more, and much of it is an unwanted burden and responsibility. It's good to see what we can give away, rather than what we can acquire or hang on to. Material things are good gifts of God to be used and enjoyed, but our real treasure is laid up for us in Heaven where nothing can damage or steal it (Luke 12:34).

Prevailing prayers

As we approach old age, many of us will have prayed for many years, sometimes with tears and groanings, for those of our children, grandchildren, family and friends who do not yet know the Lord, or for situations that have not yet been resolved. We may have become weary in this intercession, felt like giving up, or that our prayers are not heard or that God will not answer.

Take heart. God hears. He sees (and collects) our tears, he knows the deep desires of our hearts, he hears each heartfelt intercession. Prayer is never wasted. Whenever we pray, something happens in the spiritual realm. We may not see exactly the answers we asked for when we want them, but God is at work in ways we don't dream of, in the lives of those we love. Keep praying. Even if we never see the results in this life, God is faithful and will surely answer in his own way and his own time (1 Corinthians 1:9).

Promises of God (for old age)

God has wonderful promises for the aged, and meditating on these Scriptures will lift us up in body, mind and spirit.

Joel 2:28
Psalm 71
Psalm 92:14
Jeremiah 31:13
Psalm 56:12
Psalm 91:16
Psalm 86:11-15
Psalm 103:5
Isaiah 40:31
Romans 8
Philippians 4:6-7

There are many more.

qQ

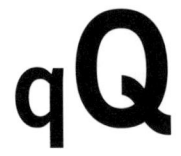

Quarrels

See also
Forgiveness

Nothing is sadder than a quarrel that has not been mended and forgiven, and has been allowed to continue and fester for years. It hurts the other person or persons, but if we are the one who can't forgive it will hurt us most of all.

Let's do our utmost to reach out and mend quarrels and differences, even if we've been badly hurt or know that we're the one in the right. It mightn't be easy, but God will help us and will take away the bitterness and hardness if we ask him.

Querulousness

See also
Mellowing

There are plenty of querulous old folks around, so we don't want to add to their numbers by becoming critical or complaining ourselves, however justified we feel it to be. God by his spirit can give us a sweetness and a kindness that will draw people and bless them rather than making them want to avoid us.

rR

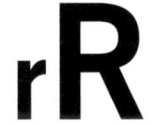

Reading
See **Books, Glasses**

Regrets
See also **Forgiveness, Quarrels**

It's sometimes tempting, looking back over the years, to give in to feelings of regret – for opportunities missed, wrong decisions made, things done (and said) that shouldn't have been, things left undone that should. Everyone has regrets. The thing to do with them is hand them over to God, ask forgiveness if necessary, and then refuse to spend more time and energy regretting what might have been. We have a God who is in the business of restoration, even of the 'years which the locust has eaten'.

Relinquishment

There can be a real sense of loss that comes with relinquishment – particularly for those who have retired from an active career or involvement with decision-making and responsible posts and jobs. It's hard to hand over the reins, to let someone else take a lead. Ideally, an older person would be asked to contribute their wisdom and experience in other capacities, to the benefit of those coming after. If this doesn't seem to be happening, don't allow frustration and bitterness to creep in. Ask God to provide fulfilling work for you to do.

AN A-Z GUIDE TO GETTING OLDER

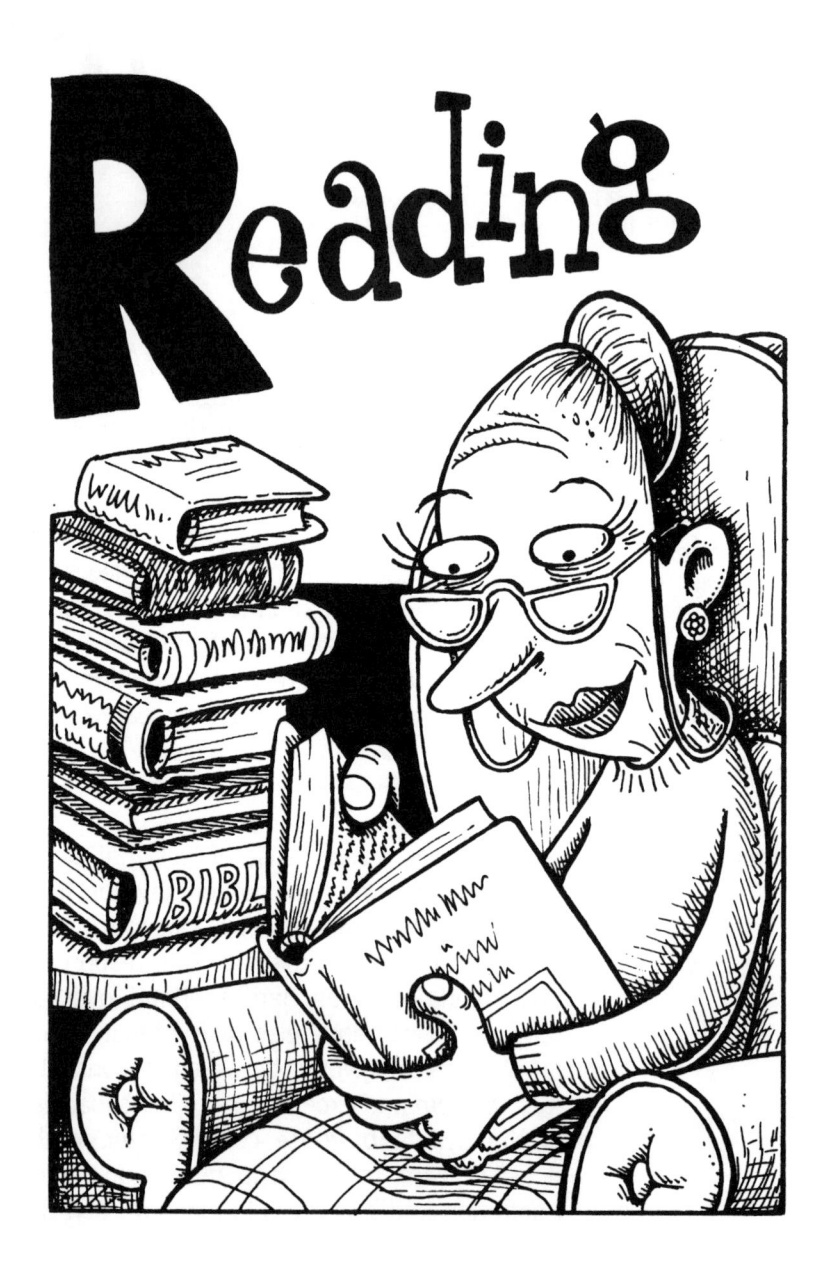

Reading

Reminiscence

See **Memories, Nostalgia**

Respect

We may feel we're not getting the respect we deserve as Senior Citizens, and we may be right. Some sectors of our society do seem to marginalise older people, and this can be deeply hurtful. Remember that in God's eyes we are every bit as valuable and precious as younger ones, and let's respect ourselves accordingly. Let's remember too to respect others, even those we don't agree with or those whose values are not our own.

Retirement

However much anticipated, retirement can sometimes not quite be what we thought it would be. This may be especially hard for us wives when our husbands retire. Suddenly, there he is, in the house and under our feet at all hours of the day. We may have looked forward to a bit more togetherness time, and be nonplussed to find that it's sometimes irritating to have him directing the shopping, peering into saucepans while we're cooking, advising us on things we've managed perfectly well for years by ourselves, or just simply 'being there' when we're used to solitude and routine.

Most couples adjust. It's good to have a few projects lined up that can be tackled together, or a holiday trip, or a new study course, or a shared ministry. Taking out the grandchildren (or travelling to visit the more distant ones) is a wonderfully fulfilling and fun way to spend the day, and their busy parents will be glad of the respite too. There are so many creative ways to make retirement a rich and positive time in your lives.

Rivalry

A rather subtle and unexpected form of rivalry can creep in when we become grandparents. Most of us will boast about the charm, beauty and accomplishments of our grandchildren to other grans and grandads – it's par for the course. More worrying, maybe, is when grandparents with more than one set of grandchildren fall into the habit of praising one set to the parents of the others, and vice versa. It's not always understood that they do just the same with the other set, and can be quite hurtful. Encourage your children by praising their children to them, affirming their own status as good parents and avoiding unnecessary jealousy.

Routine

It's reassuring to get settled into comfortable routines as we get older. Most of us don't welcome too many shake-ups or disturbances or changes. Let's not get too deep into our ruts though. Something different now and then – whether it's a food we haven't tried, another venue for Christmas, asking new friends for a meal, or getting up an hour earlier to go for a walk – will help keep us fresh and young.

S

Saga

Saga is an organisation for those aged 50 and over, providing holidays, products and services at discounted prices. For more information contact: Saga Holidays Ltd, FREEPOST (FO49), Folkstone, Kent. CT20 3ZH.
 Or visit the Saga website on www.saga.co.uk

Saying no

Sometimes it seems that younger people (maybe family members) are determined to organise their elders, find things to occupy them, clubs to join, projects for them to get involved with. This is all well and good, but no one should feel obliged to take up everything they're offered, or help with every special event (even Christian ones!) Everyone should be free to say no, when they need to, without feeling ungrateful or guilty.

Scriptures

See also
**Bible Study,
Promises of God**

Studying and searching the Scriptures, meditating upon them, and memorising Scripture verses is something that's vital to us throughout our lives and into our later years. There's always fresh truth to be found in the riches of God's inspired word, new strengths and insights to be integrated into our lives. We'll find that words

AN A-Z GUIDE TO GETTING OLDER

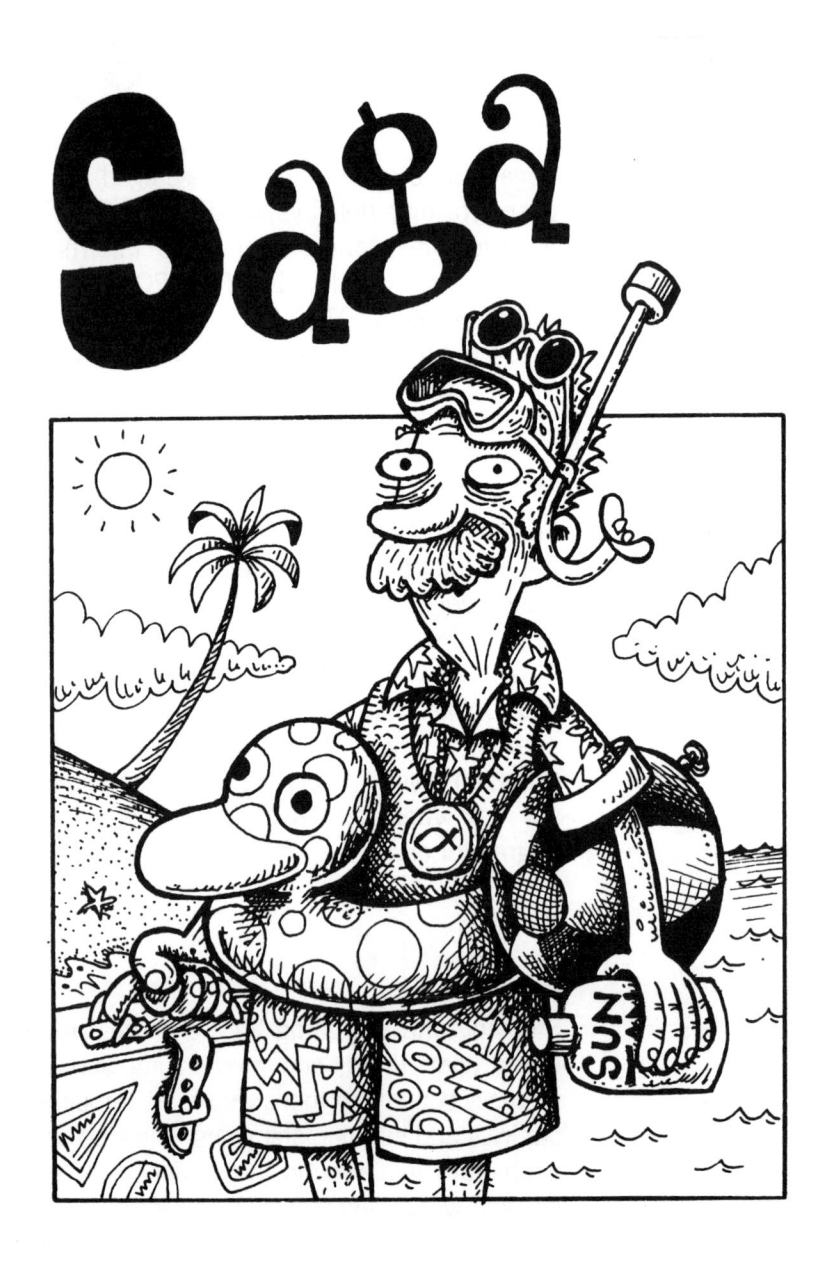

Saga

and passages will often come into our minds at times when we need them most.

Most Bible versions are available in large print for those whose eyesight is failing, and there are Scripture tapes and cassettes that can be borrowed or hired.

Self-knowledge

One advantage of years is that we do become more self-aware, we know (to some degree at least) what makes us tick, we understand some of the influences that have made us as we are, we have learned by experience what our reactions and responses will be in given situations, or what we're capable of.

We may still find we surprise ourselves, though, with what we can achieve and accomplish with God's help. And it's a great comfort to know that we are still God's beloved children, and that he knows us through and through, whatever our age.

Set in our ways

See also
Just the two of us again, Routine

Let's not get set in too firm a mould, however comfortable. It's good to be jogged out of our comfort zones now and then and be spontaneous, act on impulse, or do something slightly out of character, however askance the younger generation may look at us. They don't have the monopoly on freshness and spontaneity.

Simplicity

See also
Possessions

A high-maintenance lifestyle with a large house and garden to keep up, expensive possessions or lots of time-consuming collections to care for is not the best option for later life. Now is maybe the time to see what can be done to simplify matters, perhaps giving away or recycling some of our 'things' and generally cutting down the clutter. There'll always be some precious things we'll want to keep, of course. But paring down, scaling down and settling for a simpler life can be great fun too, and a challenge in itself.

Sleep

See also
Bed, King-size bed, Nights

It's a fact that older people need rather less sleep, although everyone needs adequate rest. Sleep patterns may change, older people may find they sleep in spells of two or three hours at a time with wakeful periods between, rather than a seven or eight-hour stretch. A restful winding-down time before bed, with a warm bath or shower and milky drink will help encourage sleep. A spell of reading or watching TV tucked up in bed, with proper back support, can be wonderfully relaxing. And a little cat-nap in the daytime can work wonders.

Stiffness

See **Exercise, Joints**

Studying

A course of study at evening classes, the local library, college, or even university, could be just what a retired person needs to give them a sense of purpose and of being in the swing of things again. The local Education Authority will be able to give details of what's available. (There's lots.)

Apart from the interest and sense of achievement, you'll also meet new people, make new friends and be stimulated in all kinds of ways. It's never too late to learn more about something that interests you, or to master a new skill or have another string to your bow.

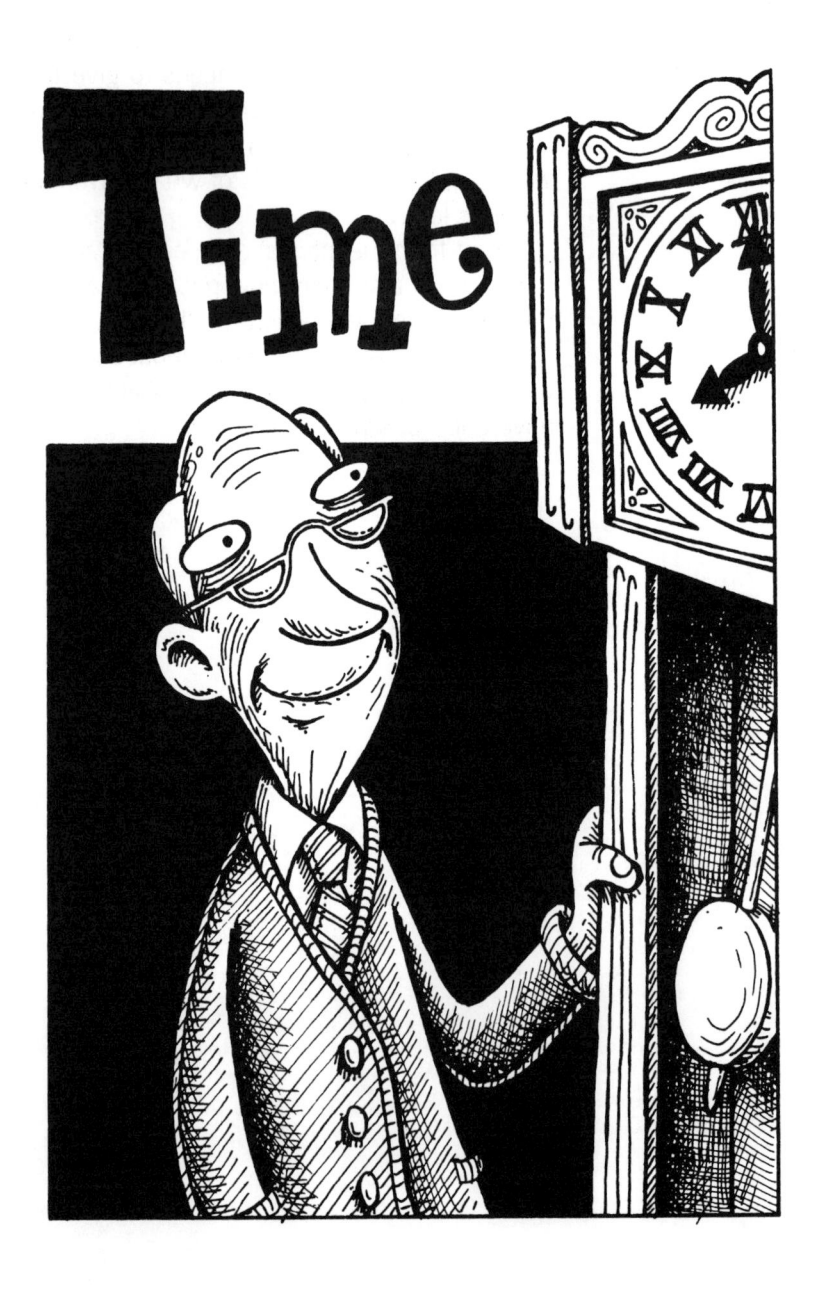

Time

T

Technology

See also
Computers, E-mail, Mobile phone

The workings of modern technology may seem like something from another planet as we get older. How many of us have had to resort to asking our grandchildren to show us how to work the video recorder, or the mobile phone or the computer? A lot of the technical talk flying around sounds like a foreign language to our ears.

It needn't be. We're perfectly capable of learning something new if we put our minds to it. It's one of the ploys of the enemy to make us feel useless, or past it, or afraid of making fools of ourselves, or that it's all beyond us. It's not.

Thanksgiving

Giving thanks to God is good, whatever our circumstances, however we're feeling. Thanksgiving helps us to focus on God, reminds us that he's in control of everything, lifts our hearts and takes our minds off ourselves.

Time

It's a strange paradox that time passes faster as we get older, even though most of us actually have more time on our hands. Maybe it has something to do with becoming more aware of our own mortality.

At every stage of life we need to use our time wisely. That doesn't mean rushing around trying to cram in everything we can, but rather that first and foremost we spend time with God, learning to know him and his will for our lives daily, to hear his voice and to obey it. God has prepared in advance the works that we are to do, and the time to do them.

Trust

Sooner or later, most Christians come to a place where they have planned, worked, prayed, and done all they can in a situation, seemingly to no avail. I'm thinking especially about children and family members who have not yet yielded their lives to God, or who need healing or deliverance of some kind. Sometimes we feel that it's all been in vain, that some things will never change.

When we feel we can do no more, it's often time to take our hands right off and turn it all over to God. It's been said that our extremity is God's opportunity. When we stop struggling and striving and trust God with the whole thing (our frantic prayers included) he will often surprise us with what happens.

Understanding

See also
Wisdom

We can never hope to understand God, whose thoughts are not our thoughts and whose ways are far above ours.

However, a long life for the Christian does bring with it the promise of a greater degree of understanding (Job 12:12).

We will be able to look back and see to some extent what God has been doing in and through our lives. We will understand better the needs of our fellow humans and of the world, and the heart of God towards them.

vV

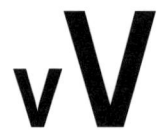

Values

Our values will change as we age. We'll no longer have the usual ambitions that inspire younger people – success in studies, training and work, the founding of a happy marriage and family, promotion, etc. Most of us will find our horizons narrowing and our needs more modest – at least in the physical and material sense. In the spiritual, the sky is still the limit and as Christians our hearts are still firmly fixed on the values of God's kingdom; values which are not always those of the world.

Visiting

With more time on our hands, visiting can be a most fulfilling ministry of the later years. There are all kinds of people – and not just older ones – who would welcome a visitor. Young mums, disabled or housebound people, newcomers to the area, singles living alone – all might be more inclined to welcome a visit from a friendly, non-threatening, relaxed older person, than they would to go to church. Don't feel rebuffed if there are some who plainly don't want visitors. Pray for the folk you meet, take an interest and get to know and accept them, warts and all, and realise that they are people whom God loves and wants to draw closer to himself – maybe through you.

Voluntary work

Voluntary work does seem to be mostly the prerogative of the older and retired people among us. How many charity shops, drop-in centres, coffee shops, church events, bookstalls – to name but a few – would survive and thrive if not for the oldies? Voluntary work is a jolly good way of staying in the swim of things and getting to know people.

Don't overdo it though. Most voluntary work shifts are for half a day, morning or afternoon, and by the end of the shift, you'll probably need, and deserve, a nice cup of tea with your feet up.

wW

Weight

It's not good to be much overweight at any age, and as both men and women get older, the weight does seem to go on more easily and stick more stubbornly. Obesity is a contributory factor to many illnesses, and is best avoided. A sensible diet, with plenty of fresh fruit and veg, wholegrain cereals and non-fatty meat and fish, combined with regular exercise, will go a long way to keeping weight under control.

Wills

See also
Money, Plans

Making a will is a sensible step and need not be complicated. It's vital to do it properly and legally though. Changes can be added later if necessary. A will can relieve much of the strain from a newly-bereaved family.

Wisdom

See also
Understanding

There's nothing more comforting and reassuring to a troubled younger person than a wise, experienced older person to whom they can go for counsel and guidance. Most people do gain through a lifetime's experience, though not all will become mines of information or founts of wisdom.

The best wisdom is that gained from a lifetime's close walk with God, from familiarity with the Scriptures as a guidebook, and from communicating with God by prayer and listening. With such wisdom, an older person really has something to offer those in need.

Work

See also
Voluntary work

There is absolutely no need for anyone to feel they're useless, redundant or have nothing to contribute to the community just because they're retired or older. There's always work to do in the Kingdom of God! Even for the housebound or disabled, ministries abound. Letter writing can be one of the most rewarding of ministries – there are Christians in prisons, in this country and abroad, for example, who rely on letters from other Christians for their support and fellowship. There are children in sponsorship programmes in the Third World who can blossom and grow with the help of letters; to missionaries and others far from home a letter is a lifeline and a great encouragement.

An older person is often invaluable when it comes to leading prayer groups and the like – offering their homes for gatherings, or being available to people like young marrieds, or mums and toddlers who may be far from their own families and in need of some loving advice or common sense, or just a cup of tea and chat. A family at church may need a 'substitute gran' to keep an eye on a schoolchild for an hour or two until their parents finish work. Another elderly person or couple might be glad to share a meal and fellowship from time to time. You could offer to change someone's library book. Or walk their dog. Or offer them a lift to and from church, and so on.

Worry

Some people worry more than others. With some, worry is almost a habit, their first reaction when anything goes wrong with a child, or a family member, or at home or work or church.

As we age, the worry can become focused upon ourselves. Most of the other concerns are someone else's responsibility now. But our own concerns – our health, or our circumstances or decisions about our future – can loom very large in our minds.

Now, as ever, God is there inviting us to cast all our cares upon him. He tells us not to be anxious, but with thanksgiving to bring our needs before him (Philippians 4:6).

He promises to care for us into our old age. And he tells us that he will never, never, leave us or forsake us (Psalm 37:25).

Worship

Different churches and individuals may have different ideas about worship. Often there seem to be separate worship services for different age-groups – maybe it's thought that older people can't put up with the noise the younger ones seem to relish so much!

The best worship is when all ages – from babies to pensioners – are worshipping together, forgetting their differences because God is at the centre of their worship; and in focusing on him in praise and adoration, age ceases to have meaning.

Wrinkles

Wrinkles happen as the skin ages and loses its elasticity, and the layer of fat under the skin changes. Some are more wrinkle-free than others. It's possible to spend a small fortune on anti-wrinkle creams and potions, even more on facelifts and tucks and so on. How much more restful to accept ourselves as we are, with all the lines and folds that a lifetime of living, loving, laughter, tears and sunshine has brought us.

Writing

See also
Journalising

In keeping a diary, journal, or some other account of our lives and times we can lay up a goldmine of interest and information to those who will come after us. Letters, notes and postcards – even household accounts and shopping lists – can piece together and bring to life a day and age that is past and gone – though it would probably take a whole room to store all that paperwork! I may not leave much money to my descendants, but I intend to write as long as I can hold a pen, and hope that some of them will appreciate the flavour of the era, the changing seasons, the family details and the happenings and events that took place in my lifetime.

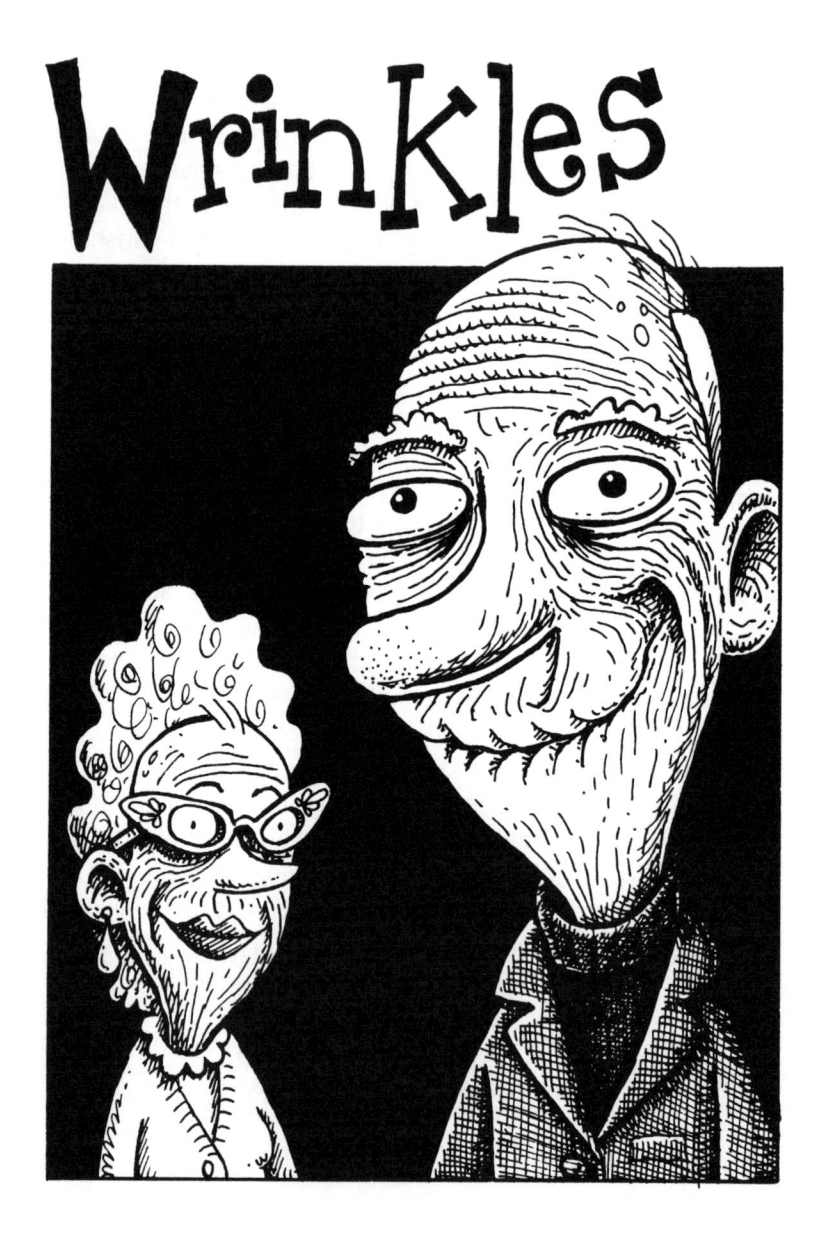

Wrinkles

xX

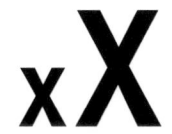

X – the unknown factor

All of us wonder about the unknown, and maybe as we get older we think more about death, the great unknown.

As Christians, we believe that death will be merely a new beginning, the beginning of a wonderful eternity with God. We can look back over our lifespan, and seeing how God has kept us and cared for us, we can safely trust him to take us through to the very ends of our lives here and into the next.

yY

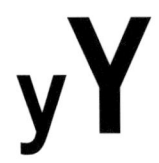

Young people

Skipping a generation is often a good recipe for getting on well! Many young people feel they can confide in their grandparents (or others of their grandparents' generation) in a way that they can't with their parents. A step removed, older people are often less judgemental and more understanding than those directly responsible. The older ones often very much enjoy the company of youngsters, appreciate their openness and up-front attitudes, learn much about the world as seen through their eyes, and even learn to like their vocabulary and their music (if only in small doses!)

Youth

See also
Promises of God

God has wonderful promises for us as we travel on through life and into the later years. The best news is that, inside, we need never grow old, because he has actually promised to renew our youth day by day (Isaiah 40:31).

zZ

Zest

Someone who has a real zest for life, who enjoys each day to the full, who makes the most of every opportunity and is enthusiastic and positive, is an attractive person whatever their age. Let's not sit about feeling our lives are over (or the best part of them) or feeling sorry for ourselves as we age. With God's help, let's determine to keep our zest, our sparkle, our joy, as we run the final lap of the course that's been set out for us, looking forward to even greater delights beyond (1 Corinthians 9:24-25).

A prayer for later life

Dear Father God,

Thank you for the long years of the life you have given, for its joys and its sorrows, its triumphs and failures, its gains and its losses. Thank you for the blessings of families, of work, of the richness of friendships, of the variety of the changing seasons and of the world we live in. Thank you most of all for your presence with us, and for the joy of a growing and developing relationship with you through your son Jesus. Thank you for the blood of Jesus that cleanses and covers all of our failures and shortcomings. Thank you for your Holy Spirit who lives in us.

Help us now to live with courage and joy the rest of the time we have here on earth, welcoming each day as a new gift from you. Help us to depend on your word, to lean on your strength, to trust you in all situations that arise. Thank you that you have gone before us to prepare our place in Heaven, and that soon we will meet you face to face.
Amen